Superfood Seamoss Smoothies

SHAWNTE PARKS - NATURAL VEGAN MAMA
AUTHOR OF PRETTY LADIES EAT PLANTS
PALM BEACH COUNTY, FLORIDA

Health is the thing that
makes you feel that now is
the best time of the year.

FRAKLIN P. ADAMS

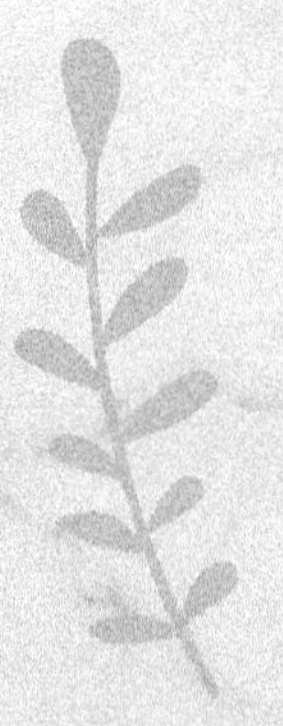

Recipes
all recipes are one serving unless stated otherwise..

Crazy Cucumber 1

Kickin' Kiwi 2

Always Avocado 3

Anytime Apple 4

Make it Matcha 5

Kind Kale 6

Help Me Hemp 7

Bangin' Banana 8

Seriously Seedy 9

totally turmeric 10

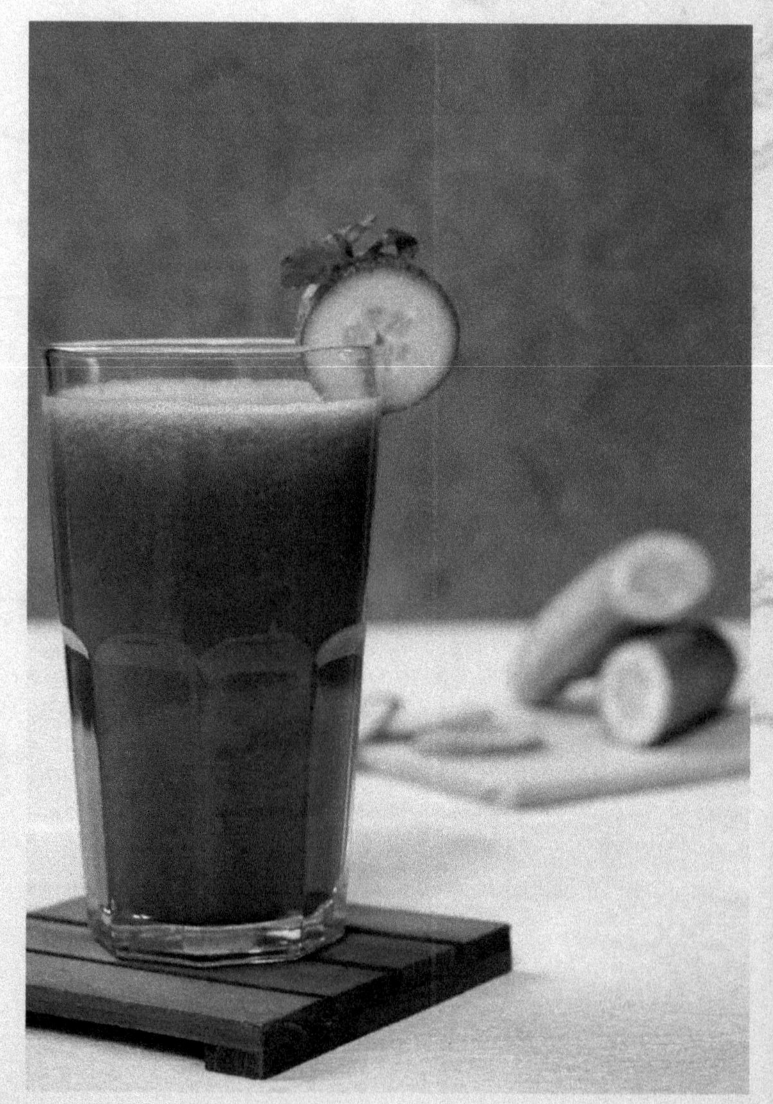

Crazy Cucumber

2 cups spinach
1 cup chopped cucumber
1 cup chopped pineapple
1 tablespoon sea moss gel
8oz spring water

blend

garnish with cucumber and mint

enjoy

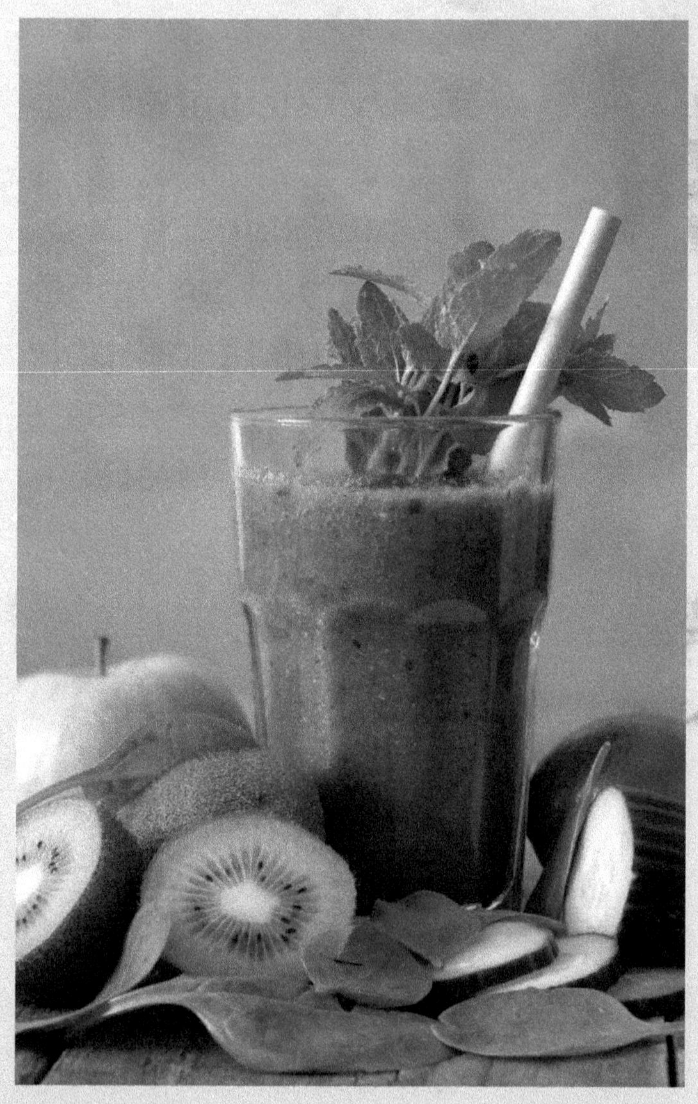

Kickin' Kiwi

2 cups kale
1 cup chopped kiwi
1 green apple
1/2 cup cucumber
1 tablespoon sea moss gel
8oz spring water

blend

garnish with kiwi and mint

enjoy

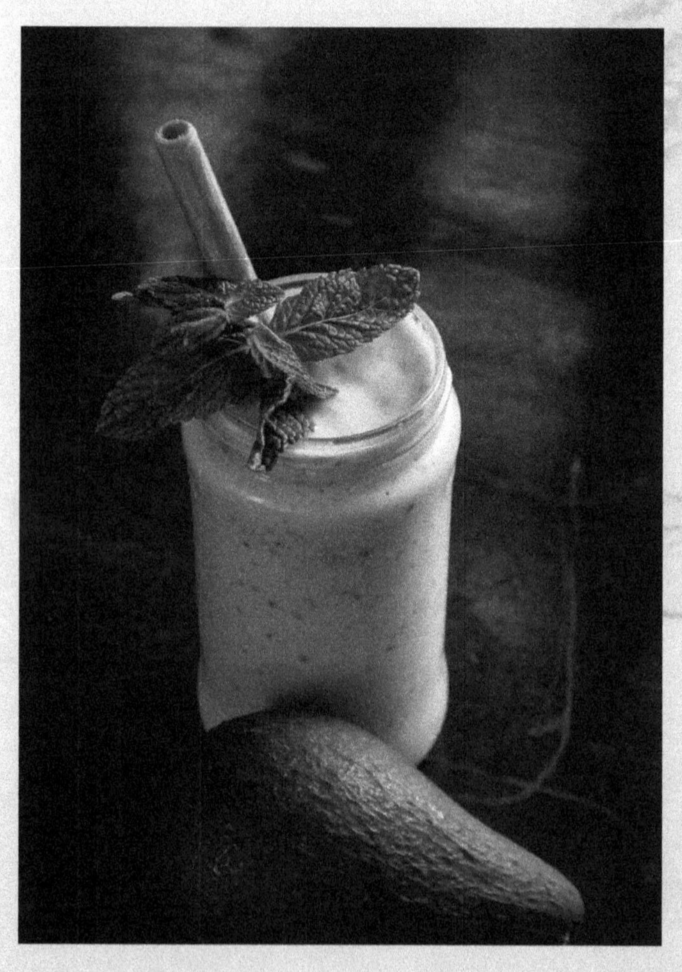

Always Avocado

2 cups spinach
1 avocado
1/2 frozen banana
1 tablespoon sea moss gel
8oz spring water

blend

garnish with mint

enjoy

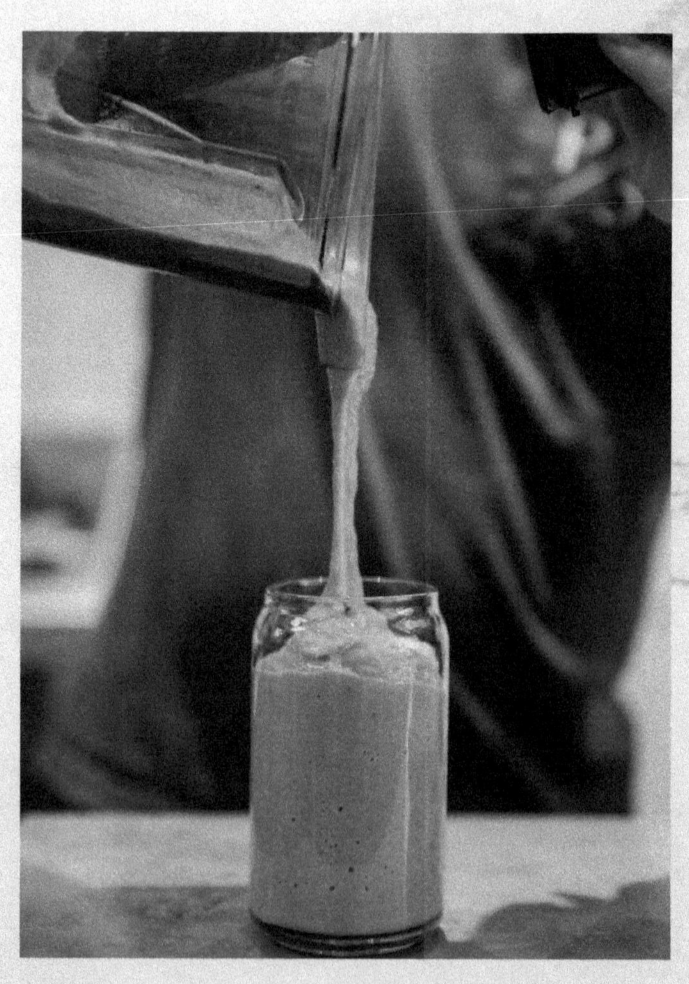

Always Apple

2 cups spinach
1 green apple
1 cup frozen banana
1 tablespoon sea moss gel
8 oz spring water

blend

garnish with mint

enjoy

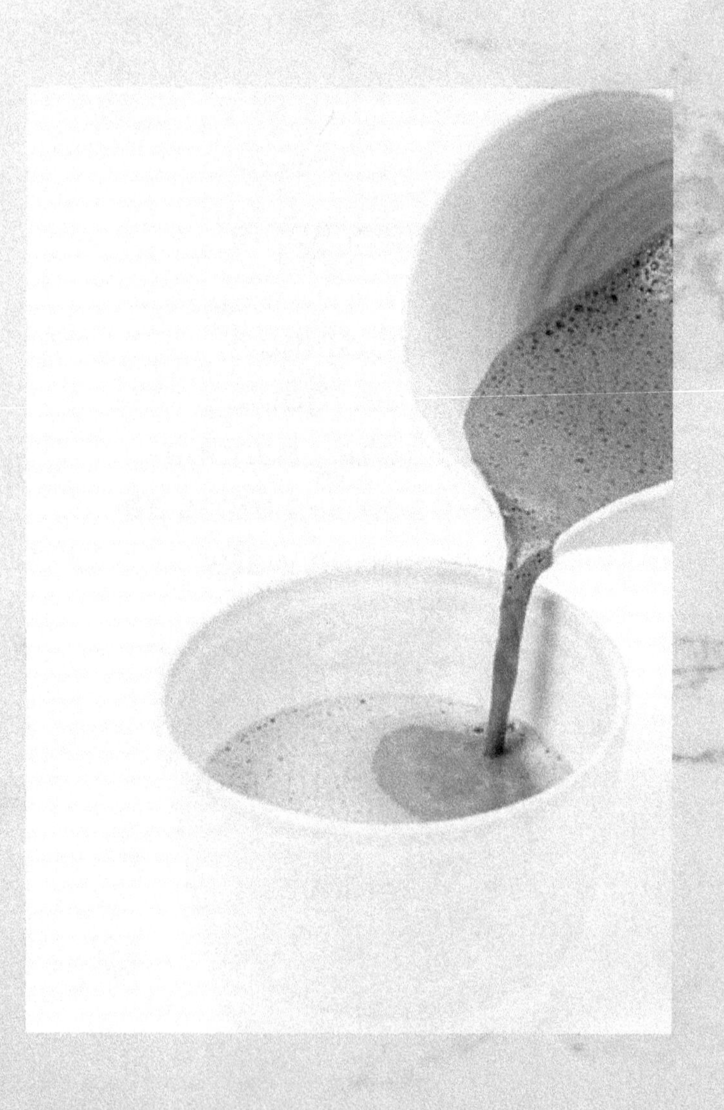

Make It Matcha

2 cups spinach
1 teaspoon matcha powder
1/2 frozen banana
1 tablespoon sea moss gel
8 oz spring water

blend

garnish with mint

enjoy

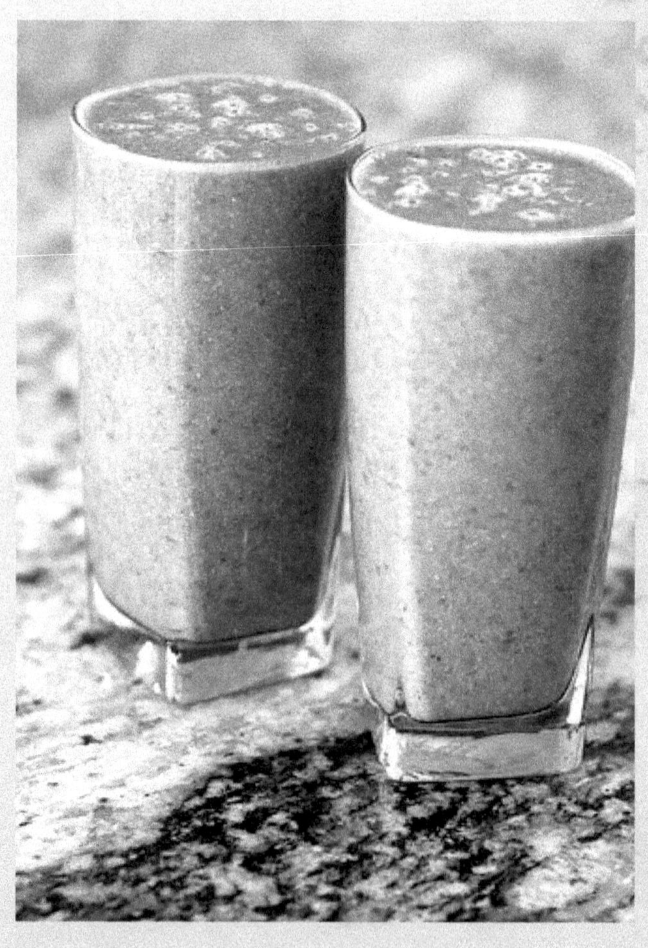

Kind Kale
2 servings

2 cups kale
1 green apple
1 cup frozen banana
2 tablespoons sea moss gel
16 oz spring water

blend

garnish with mint

enjoy

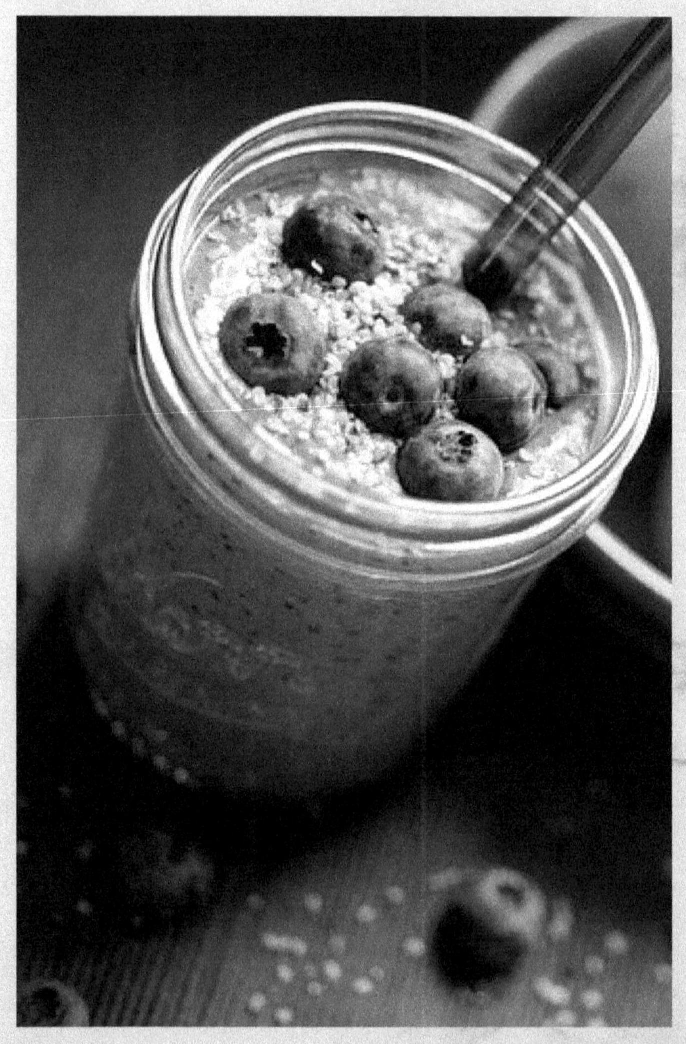

Help Me Hemp

2 cups spinach
1 cup blueberries
1/2 avocado
1 tablespoon sea moss gel
1 tablespoon hemp seeds
8 oz spring water

blend

garnish with mint

enjoy

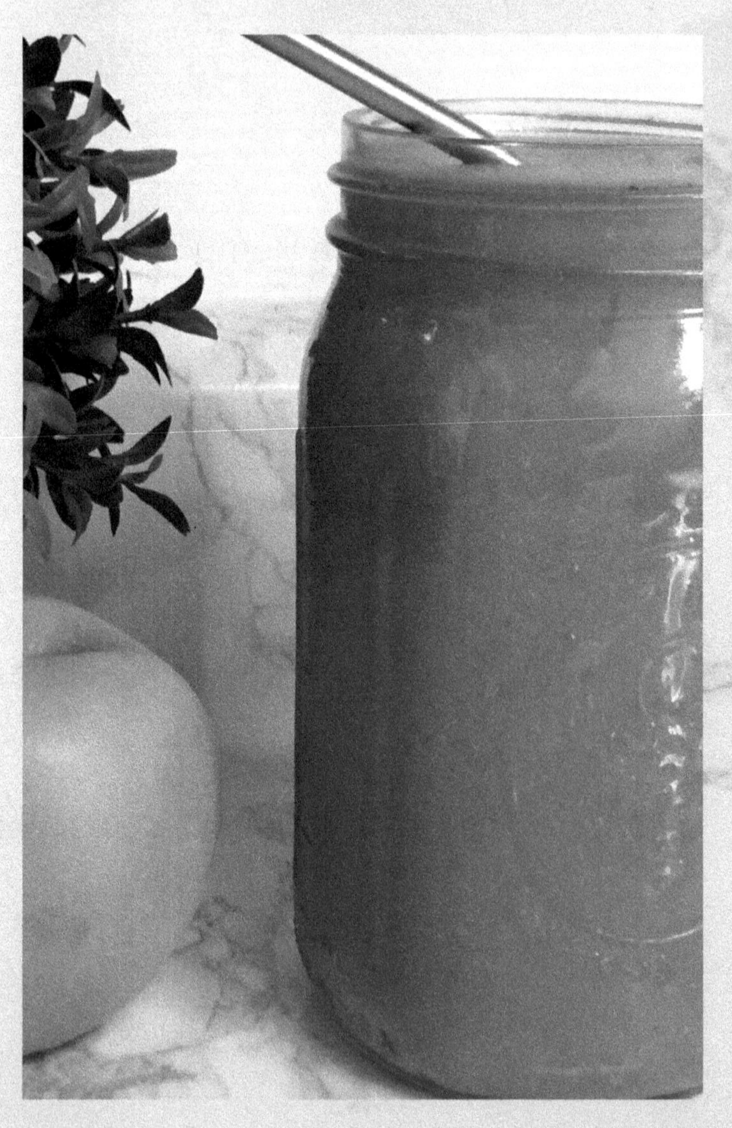

Bangin' Banana

2 cups spinach
1 cup kale
1 frozen banana
1 tablespoon sea moss gel
1 green apple
8 oz spring water

blend

garnish with mint

enjoy

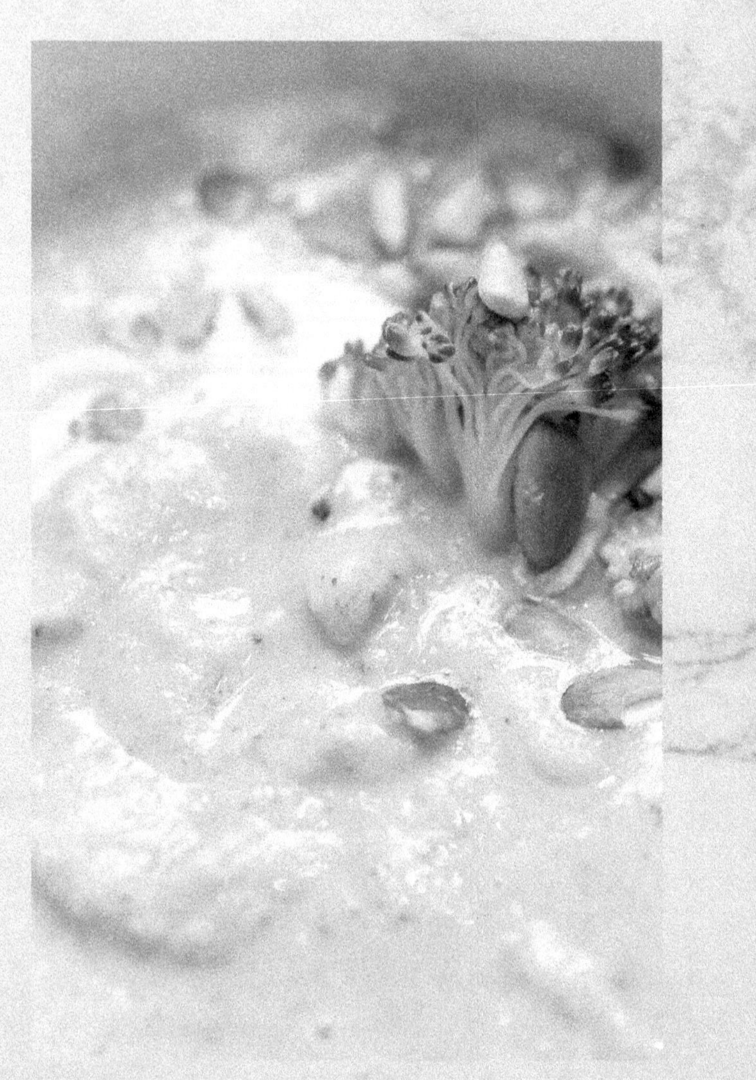

Seriously Seedy

2 cups spinach
1 cup kale
1/2 cup broccoli
1 tablespoon sea moss gel
1 teaspoon sunflower seeds
1 teaspoon pumpkin seeds
8 oz spring water

blend

garnish with 1 broccoli floret,
1/2 tsp sunflower seeds and
1/2 teaspoon pumpkin seeds

enjoy

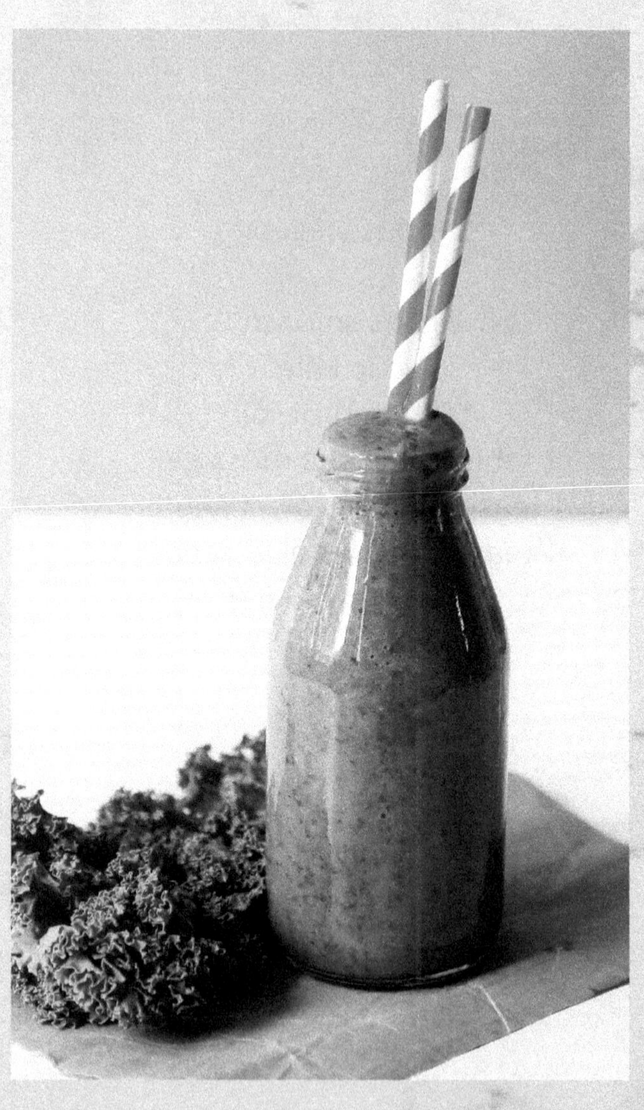

Totally Turmeric

2 cups spinach
1 cup kale
1 teaspoon turmeric
1 cup frozen mango
1 tablespoon sea moss gel
8 oz spring water

blend

garnish with mint

enjoy

ALSO AVAILABLE ON AMAZON..

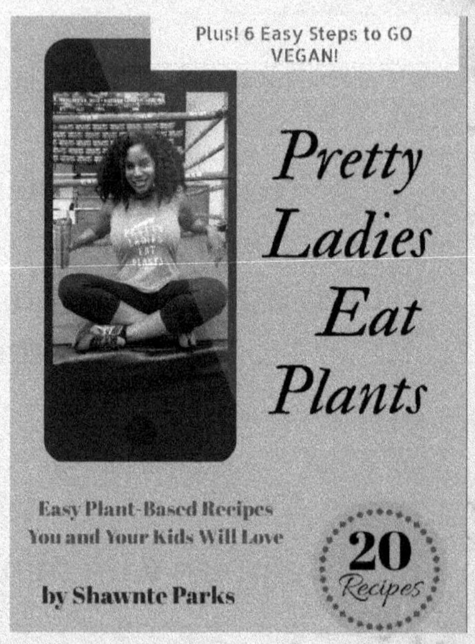

Thank you for your
purchase.
If you enjoyed this recipe
book
please leave a review!
Follow me for more recipes

Natural Vegan Mama

 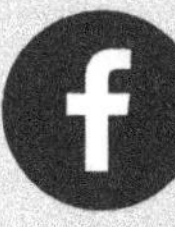 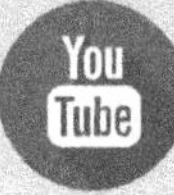

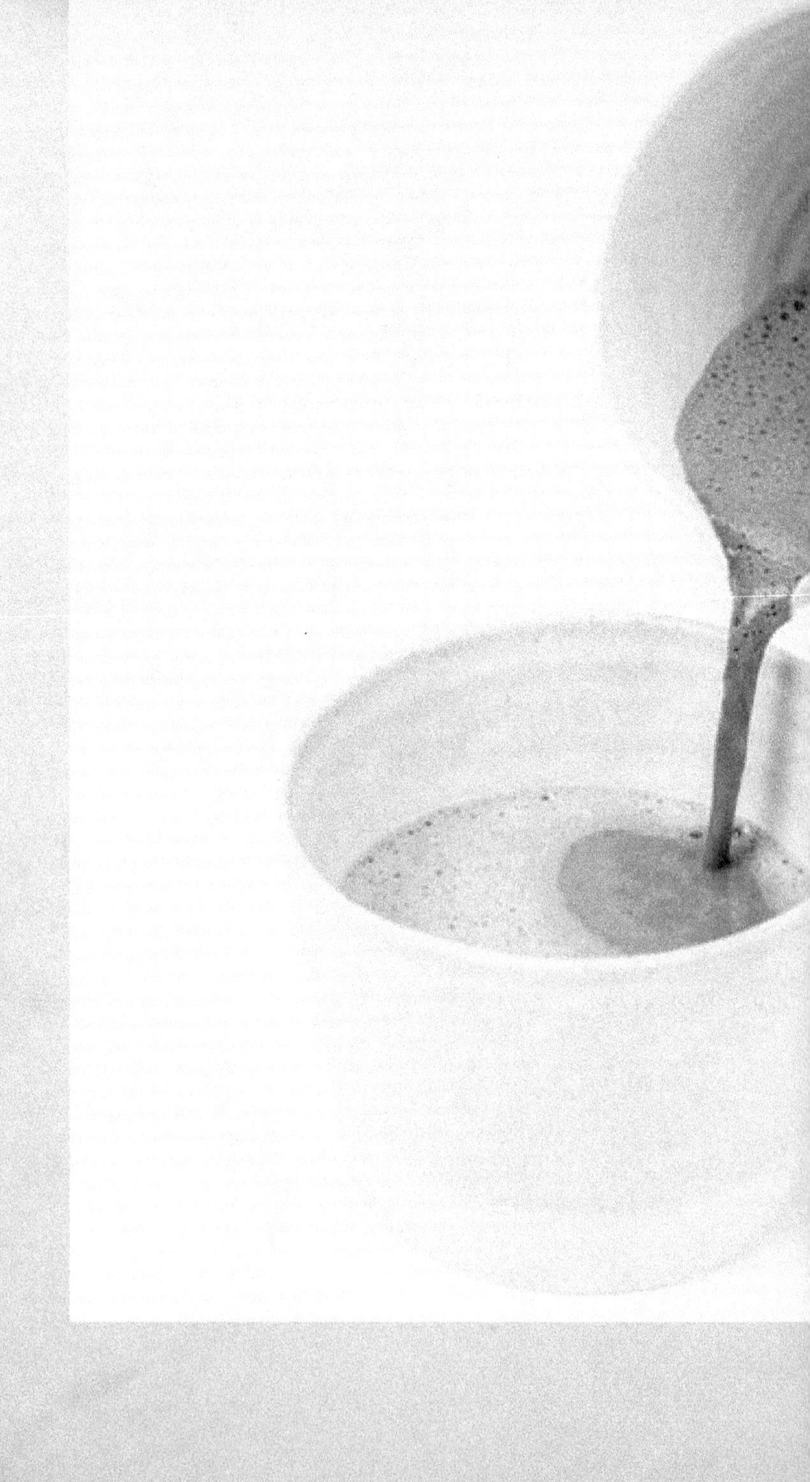